21 Day Home Boot Camp Workout

Get Fit And Drop A Dress Or Pant Size In Just 30 Minutes A Day!

© 2012 Kris Crepeau

Disclaimer: No part of this book may be used or reproduced in any manner whatsoever without written permission except in the case of brief quotations utilized in articles and reviews. The programs and information expressed within this book are not medical advice, but rather represent the author's opinions and are solely for informational and educational purposes. The author is not responsible in any manner whatsoever for any injury or health condition that may occur through following the programs and opinions expressed herein. Dietary information is presented for informational purposes only and may not be appropriate for all individuals. Consult with your physician before starting any exercise program or altering your diet.

Table of Contents

About The Author

Kris Crepeau is a Certified Personal Trainer, Author, and Entrepreneur. He has created numerous fitness websites, apps, and written many books. Kris has a passion for fitness and creating workouts that help people live a fit and healthy lifestyle.

Introduction

Drop the extra pounds and tighten and tone those trouble areas in just 30 minutes a day. Don't be fooled, it's only 30 minutes but it's not an easy workout by any means. You will be challenged at any fitness level, but the workout is designed with timed intervals so you can progress at your own pace. Whether you can do 5 or 25 pushups to start you can improve on your numbers with each workout, but don't get caught up in the numbers. Quality not quantity, make sure you are doing each rep of each exercise in good form and stop when you can no longer perform the exercise with good form. You might find if you find yourself losing good form and if you rest for a few seconds you might be able to get a couple more reps in with good form. Included in this book are pictures and descriptions of the 60 exercises that are part of this workout.

This workout is not meant to be a long term workout solution. It is however a perfect solution if you:

- Want to drop a dress or pant size for a wedding or an upcoming vacation
- Are tired of going to the gym and not seeing results
- Are tired of boring workouts like running on the treadmill for an hour
- Have hit a plateau in your usual workout routine
- Plan on joining a local fitness boot camp program and would like to get familiar with some of the exercises and training style
- Need a jumpstart to getting involved in some type of fitness program

What Is A Boot Camp workout?

A Boot Camp workout is based around the basic concept of a military callisthenic workout. While today's modern fitness boot camp workouts incorporate everything from kettlebells to battle ropes, the idea is built around a fast paced total body workout with little rest in between exercises.

What Should I Eat?

I'm not going to go too in depth here about nutrition, but this workout will not get you the results you are looking for if you don't eat right. Where most people go wrong is not planning ahead what you're going to eat. Do yourself a favor and just grab a blank piece of paper and plan out your meals for the next 21 days (it won't kill you, I promise) Most people eat pretty much the same things every few days so it's not like you have to make all 21 days completely different. Plan out Breakfast, Lunch, Dinner, and Snacks.

You don't have to go crazy to make a significant difference in the foods you eat. Start out by cutting out obvious things like fried foods and pastries. Next substitute processed snacks like granola bars and 100 calorie pack mini muffins with a bag of nuts or fresh fruit and vegetables. You'd be surprised at how much more full you'll get when you add in more fruits and vegetables into your diet as snacks and with your meals. The bottom line (pun intended) is eat more whole foods, fruits, and vegetables and cut out the fried, processed, saturated animal fat foods. If you eat better you'll feel better and you'll augment your results of any fitness program.

About the 21 Day Home Boot Camp Workout Program

This 21 Day Home Boot Camp Workout will incorporate almost exclusively no equipment exercises. The only pieces of equipment you will need are a chair and a pull up bar. You can pick up a door mounted pull up bar that mounts at the top of your door frame without having to permanently installing it. It slips on in 2 seconds and you can pick one up almost anywhere for $20 or less. As far as bodyweight exercises go, there is no other exercise that will strengthen your back like the pull up. The only other thing you'll need is something to keep time for your intervals. You can use a stop watch, timer on your wristwatch, or there are a ton of apps for your smartphone with interval timers as well.

The workout is broken up into 2 parts:

1. **Strength Workout** - Monday, Wednesday, Friday
   5 Minute Warm Up – 5 Exercises performed for 60 seconds each
   20 Minute Workout – 10 Exercises performed in order then repeat
   50/10 Intervals Monday and Friday - Perform each exercise for 50 seconds then rest for 10
   40/20 intervals on Wednesday - Perform each exercise for 40 seconds then rest for 20
   5 minute Abs/Core – 5 Exercises performed for 60 seconds each

2. **Cardio Workout** - Tuesday, Thursday, Saturday
   Burpees followed by HIIT Training

Sunday will be your rest day but that does not mean total rest, you still need to be active. Take a long walk with the kids, play some pick up basketball, just don't sit on the couch and watch tv.

The Workout

Week 1

Monday (Strength)

Warm Up:

Perform each exercise for 60 seconds with no rest in between exercises:

High Knees
Jog in place
Jumping Jacks
Arm Circles
Dynamic Arm Stretch

Main Workout:

Perform all 10 exercises in 50/10 Intervals (50 seconds of exercise and 10 seconds of rest) After completing all 10 exercises in order, repeat again so you have performed all 10 exercises twice:

Walking Lunges
Standard Push Up
Bodyweight Squat
Chair Dip
Burpee
Standard Pull Up
Step Back Lunge
Steam Engine
Divebomber Push Up
Prisoner Squat

Core/Abs:

Perform each exercise for 60 seconds with no rest in between exercises:

Side Plank Hold Left
Side Plank Hold Right
Bicycles
Plank
Superman

Finish Up with light static stretching

Tuesday (Cardio)

Start with 20 Burpees in quickest time possible with good form

Warm up with 5 minutes on Treadmill, Bike, Elliptical, or Jogging. Walking or light pedaling pace for 5 minutes.

Again choose Treadmill, Bike, Elliptical, or Jogging/Running for HIIT.

Sprinting pace at 90% effort for 30 seconds and then slow down to walking pace for 60 seconds repeat 12-15 times.

Finish up with 5 minutes of slow walking pace on Treadmill, Bike, etc.

Wednesday (Strength)

Warm Up:

Perform each exercise for 60 seconds with no rest in between exercises:

High Knees
Jog in place
Jumping Jacks

Arm Circles
Huggers

Main Workout:

Perform all 10 exercises in 40/20 Intervals (40 seconds of exercise and 20 seconds of rest) After completing all 10 exercises in order, repeat again so you have performed all 10 exercises twice:

Calf Raise Squat
Plank Push Up
Side to Side Lunge
Inchworm
Wide Grip Pull Up
Ski Jumps
Military Push Up
Deadlift Squat
Burpee
Jump Knee Tuck

Core/Abs:

Perform each exercise for 60 seconds with no rest in between exercises:

Scissors
Flutter Kicks
Boat
Torso Twist and Hold Left
Torso Twist and Hold Right

Finish Up with light static stretching

Thursday (Cardio)

Start with 20 Burpees in quickest time possible with good form

Warm up with 5 minutes on Treadmill, Bike, Elliptical, or Jogging. Brisk walking or light pedaling pace for 5 minutes.

Again choose Treadmill, Bike, Elliptical, or Jogging/Running for HIIT.

Sprinting pace at 90% effort for 30 seconds and then slow down to walking pace for 60 seconds repeat 12-15 times.

Finish up with 5 minutes of slow walking pace on Treadmill, Bike, etc.

Friday (Strength)

Warm Up:

Perform each exercise for 60 seconds with no rest in between exercises:

High Knees
Jog in place
Jumping Jacks
Arm Circles
Huggers

Main Workout:

Perform all 10 exercises in 50/10 Intervals (50 seconds of exercise and 10 seconds of rest) After completing all 10 exercises in order, repeat again so you have performed all 10 exercises twice:

Mountain Climbers
Plank Push Up
Side to Side Jumps
Bear Crawls
Decline Push Up
Lunge and Reach

Burpee with Push Up
Jump Squats
Standard Pull Up
Diamond Push Up

Core/Abs:

Perform each exercise for 60 seconds with no rest in between exercises:

Bicycles
Windshield Wipers
V Ups
Side Plank Hold Left
Side Plank Hold Right

Finish Up with light static stretching

Saturday (Cardio)

Start with 20 Burpees in quickest time possible with good form

Warm up with 5 minutes on Treadmill, Bike, Elliptical, or Jogging. Brisk walking or light pedaling pace for 5 minutes.

Again choose Treadmill, Bike, Elliptical, or Jogging/Running for HIIT.

Sprinting pace at 90% effort for 30 seconds and then slow down to walking pace for 60 seconds repeat 12-15 times.

Finish up with 5 minutes of slow walking pace on Treadmill, Bike, etc.

Week 2

Monday (Strength)

Warm Up:

Perform each exercise for 60 seconds with no rest in between exercises:

High Knees
Jog in place
Jumping Jacks
Arm Circles
Huggers

Main Workout:

Perform all 10 exercises in 50/10 Intervals (50 seconds of exercise and 10 seconds of rest) After completing all 10 exercises in order, repeat again so you have performed all 10 exercises twice:

Bodyweight Squat
Side to Side Push Up
Chair Pose
Close Grip Pull Up
Burpee
Deadlift Squat
Pike Press
Broad Jump
Spiderman Push Up
3 Position Lunge

Core/Abs:

Perform each exercise for 60 seconds with no rest in between exercises:

Side Plank Hold Left
Side Plank Hold Right

Bicycles
Plank
Superman

Finish Up with light static stretching

Tuesday (Cardio)

Start with 30 Burpees in quickest time possible with good form

Warm up with 5 minutes on Treadmill, Bike, Elliptical, or Jogging. Brisk walking or light pedaling pace for 5 minutes.

Again choose Treadmill, Bike, Elliptical, or Jogging/Running for HIIT.

Sprinting pace at 90% effort for 20 seconds and then slow down to walking pace for 20 seconds repeat 10-12 times.

Finish up with 5 minutes of slow walking pace on Treadmill, Bike, etc.

Wednesday (Strength)

Warm Up:

Perform each exercise for 60 seconds with no rest in between exercises:

High Knees
Jog in place
Jumping Jacks
Arm Circles
Huggers

Main Workout:

Perform all 10 exercises in 40/20 Intervals (40 seconds of exercise and 20 seconds of rest) After completing all 10 exercises in order, repeat again so you have performed all 10 exercises twice:

Standard Push Up
Squat Jacks
Wide Grip Pull Up
Step Back Lunge
Bear Crawl
Chair Dip
Mountain Climbers
Reverse Grip Pull Up
Wide Push Up
Super Skaters

Core/Abs:

Perform each exercise for 60 seconds with no rest in between exercises:

Scissors
Flutter Kicks
Boat
Torso Twist and Hold Left
Torso Twist and Hold Right

Finish Up with light static stretching

Thursday (Cardio)

Start with 30 Burpees in quickest time possible with good form

Warm up with 5 minutes on Treadmill, Bike, Elliptical, or Jogging. Brisk walking or light pedaling pace for 5 minutes.

Again choose Treadmill, Bike, Elliptical, or Jogging/Running for HIIT.

Sprinting pace at 90% effort for 20 seconds and then slow down to walking pace for 20 seconds repeat 10-12 times.

Finish up with 5 minutes of slow walking pace on Treadmill, Bike, etc.

Friday (Strength)

Warm Up:

Perform each exercise for 60 seconds with no rest in between exercises:

High Knees
Jog in place
Jumping Jacks
Arm Circles
Huggers

Main Workout:

Perform all 10 exercises in 50/10 Intervals (50 seconds of exercise and 10 seconds of rest) After completing all 10 exercises in order, repeat again so you have performed all 10 exercises twice:

Steam Engine
Staggered Hand Push Up
Squat Jumps
Inchworm
Lateral Leap Frog
Burpee with Push Up
Prisoner Lunges
Decline Push Up
Standard Pull Up
Jump Knee Tuck

Core/Abs:

Perform each exercise for 60 seconds with no rest in between exercises:

Bicycles
Windshield Wipers
V Ups
Side Plank Hold Left
Side Plank Hold Right

Finish Up with light static stretching

Saturday (Cardio)

Start with 30 Burpees in quickest time possible with good form

Warm up with 5 minutes on Treadmill, Bike, Elliptical, or Jogging. Brisk walking or light pedaling pace for 5 minutes.

Again choose Treadmill, Bike, Elliptical, or Jogging/Running for HIIT.

Sprinting pace at 90% effort for 20 seconds and then slow down to walking pace for 20 seconds repeat 10-12 times.

Finish up with 5 minutes of slow walking pace on Treadmill, Bike, etc.

Week 3

Monday (Strength)

Warm Up:

Perform each exercise for 60 seconds with no rest in between exercises:

High Knees
Jog in place
Jumping Jacks
Arm Circles
Huggers

Main Workout:

Perform all 10 exercises in 50/10 Intervals (50 seconds of exercise and 10 seconds of rest) After completing all 10 exercises in order, repeat again so you have performed all 10 exercises twice:

Prisoner Squats
Walking Push Ups
Deadlift Squat
Standard Pull Up
Grasshoppers
Slow Push Up
Lunge and Reach
Burpee
Wall Squat
Divebomber Push Up

Core/Abs:

Perform each exercise for 60 seconds with no rest in between exercises:

Side Plank Hold Left
Side Plank Hold Right

Bicycles
Plank
Superman

Finish Up with light static stretching

Tuesday (Cardio)

Start with 40 Burpees in quickest time possible with good form

Warm up with 5 minutes on Treadmill, Bike, Elliptical, or Jogging. Brisk walking or light pedaling pace for 5 minutes.

Again choose Treadmill, Bike, Elliptical, or Jogging/Running for HIIT.

Sprinting pace at 90% effort for 20 seconds and then slow down to walking pace for 10 seconds repeat 8-10 times.

Finish up with 5 minutes of slow walking pace on Treadmill, Bike, etc.

Wednesday (Strength)

Warm Up:

Perform each exercise for 60 seconds with no rest in between exercises:

High Knees
Jog in place
Jumping Jacks
Arm Circles
Huggers

Main Workout:

Perform all 10 exercises in 40/20 Intervals (40 seconds of exercise and 20 seconds of rest) After completing all 10 exercises in order, repeat again so you have performed all 10 exercises twice:

Walking Lunges
Crab Walk
Military Push Up
Deadlift Squat
Wide Grip Pull Up
Spiderman Push Up
3 Position Lunges
Standard Pull Up
Burpee with Push Up
Super Skaters

Core/Abs:

Perform each exercise for 60 seconds with no rest in between exercises:

Scissors
Flutter Kicks
Boat
Torso Twist and Hold Left
Torso Twist and Hold Right

Finish Up with light static stretching

Thursday (Cardio)

Start with 40 Burpees in quickest time possible with good form

Warm up with 5 minutes on Treadmill, Bike, Elliptical, or Jogging. Brisk walking or light pedaling pace for 5 minutes.

Again choose Treadmill, Bike, Elliptical, or Jogging/Running for HIIT.

Sprinting pace at 90% effort for 20 seconds and then slow down to walking pace for 10 seconds repeat 8-10 times.

Finish up with 5 minutes of slow walking pace on Treadmill, Bike, etc.

Friday (Strength)

Warm Up:

Perform each exercise for 60 seconds with no rest in between exercises:

High Knees
Jog in place
Jumping Jacks
Arm Circles
Huggers

Main Workout:

Perform all 10 exercises in 50/10 Intervals (50 seconds of exercise and 10 seconds of rest) After completing all 10 exercises in order, repeat again so you have performed all 10 exercises twice:

Step Back Lunges
Decline Push Up
Ski Jumps
Chair Dips
Calf Raise Squats
Burpee
Wide Grip Pull Up

Squat Jacks
Military Push Up
Jump Knee Tucks

Core/Abs:

Perform each exercise for 60 seconds with no rest in between exercises:

Bicycles
Windshield Wipers
V Ups
Side Plank Hold Left
Side Plank Hold Right

Finish Up with light static stretching

Saturday (Cardio)

Start with 40 Burpees in quickest time possible with good form

Warm up with 5 minutes on Treadmill, Bike, Elliptical, or Jogging. Brisk walking or light pedaling pace for 5 minutes.

Again choose Treadmill, Bike, Elliptical, or Jogging/Running for HIIT.

Sprinting pace at 90% effort for 20 seconds and then slow down to walking pace for 10 seconds repeat 8-10 times.

Finish up with 5 minutes of slow walking pace on Treadmill, Bike, etc.

Exercise Descriptions:

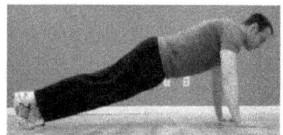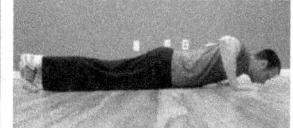

Standard Push Up - Begin with your hands and toes on the floor. Your torso and legs should remain rigid, keeping your back perfectly straight throughout the move. Bend your arms and slowly lower your body downward, stopping just before your upper chest touches the ground. Feel a stretch in your chest muscles and then reverse direction, pushing your body up along the same path back to the start position.

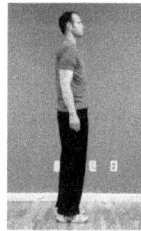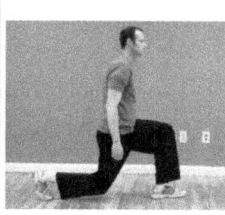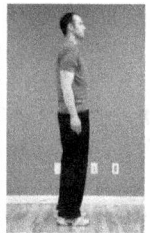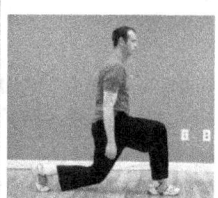

Walking Lunges – Step forward with first leg. Land on heel then forefoot. Lower body by flexing knee and hip of front leg until knee of rear leg is almost in contact with floor. Stand on forward leg with assistance of rear leg. Lunge forward with opposite leg. Repeat by alternating lunge with opposite legs.

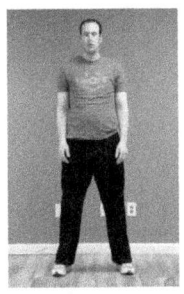 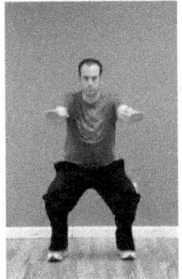

Bodyweight Squat – Stand with your feet hip-width apart, slowly lower your body down as though you were going to sit back into a chair. Keep your body weight on the heel of your foot and concentrate on sticking your hips backwards rather than just moving down. Throughout the movement keep your knees behind the line of your toes. At the lowest point your knee should be at a 90 degree angle and when you reach this point push back up to a standing position.

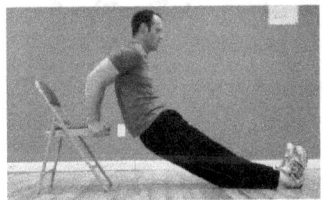 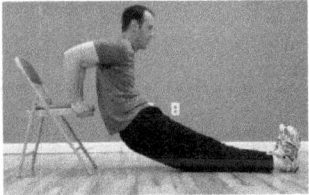

Chair Dip – Begin by placing your heels on floor and your hands on the edge of a flat bench, keeping your arms straight. Slowly bend your elbows as far as comfortably possible, allowing your butt to descend below the level of the bench. Make sure your elbows stay close to your body throughout the move. Then, reverse direction and straighten your arms, returning to the start position.

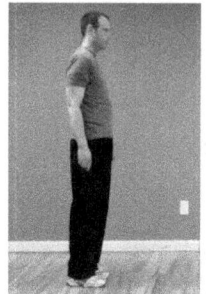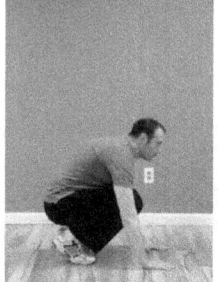
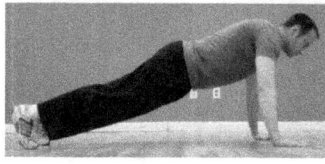

Burpee – In order to properly perform a Burpee, stand with your feet shoulder width apart with your knees slightly bent. Quickly lower your upper body until your hands touch the floor. Kick your legs out from under you and come to a normal pushup position. Hold that pose just briefly then quickly come to the position where your feet and hands are on the ground. Press back up and straighten your back. Repeat.

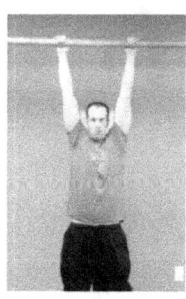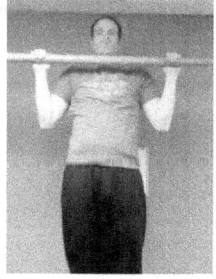

Pull Up – Begin by taking a shoulder-width, overhand grip on a chinning bar. Allow your arms to fully straighten so that you feel a complete stretch in your lats. Bend your knees and cross your ankles over one another. Keeping your back arched, slowly pull yourself upward until your chin rises above the level of the bar.

Contract your lats and then slowly lower your body back to the start position.

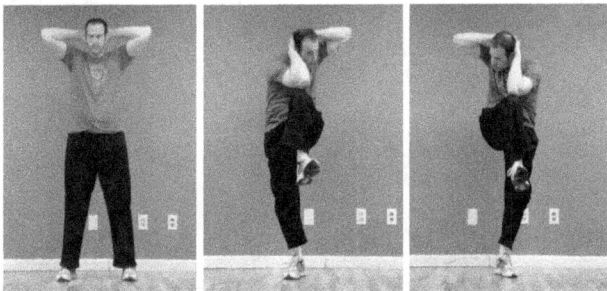

Steam Engine – Stand with your feet hip width apart and place your arms behind your neck. In a controlled manner, lift your right knee up as high as you can and bring it toward your left elbow. Pause at the top of the movement and then return your foot to the floor. Repeat the lift with your left knee to your right elbow. Continue to alternate knees.

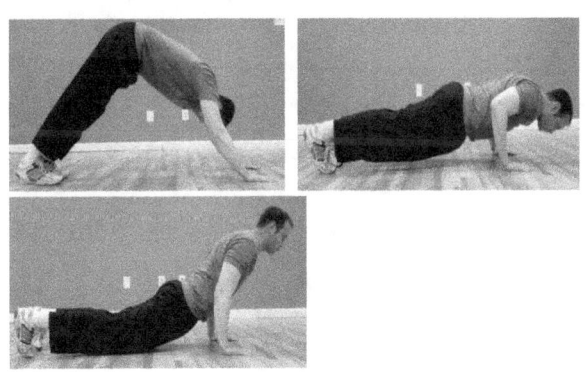

Divebomber Push Up – The dive bomber pushup starts with your hands on the floor about shoulder width or a little wider, your feet roughly shoulder width and your butt in the air. Your body looks like an inverted "V", with your head down. From that position, lower your shoulders toward the floor until your chest almost touches it, then dip your body upward. Your chest should be up, your back arched, head up and arms straight. Your pelvis rests on the floor. Hold the position for a moment and then do the movement in reverse, until you are back at the start.

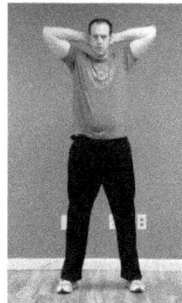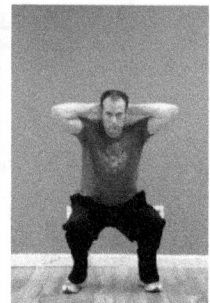

Prisoner Squat – To perform the prisoner squat stand upright with your hands crossed behind your head and your elbows back. Push your buttocks back and bend your knees as if you are going to sit down until your thighs are parallel to the floor. Don't lean forward. Contract your muscles and return to the start.

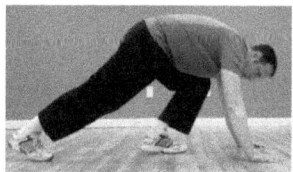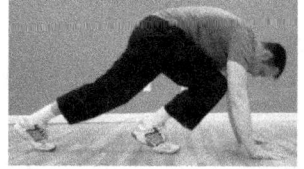

Mountain Climbers – Get in a standard push-up position. Swing your knee up to your chest then swing it back to starting position. Repeat on the other side. This movement is done quickly and is as much a cardiovascular workout as it is a strengthening exercise.

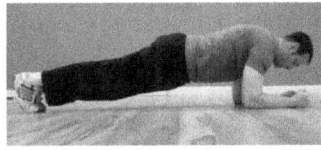 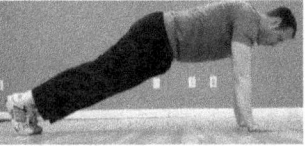

Plank Push Up – Get down into a plank position and extend your body to its full length, so that your toes are touching the floor at one end and you are resting on your forearms at the other. Your back should be fairly straight and your butt down, in line with the rest of your body. Moving one arm at a time, lift yourself up into a standard push up position. Keep your back straight and your abdominal muscles tight. Once you reach the push up position, move one arm at a time back into the starting plank position. Repeat.

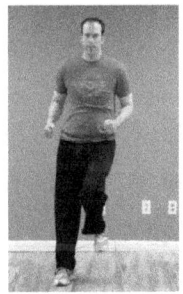 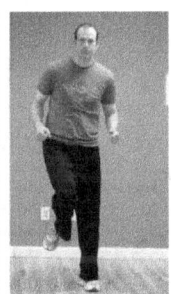

Side Jumps – Jump far to right side and land right foot with left foot off of ground. Jump far to left side landing on right foot. Continue to bound from side to side.

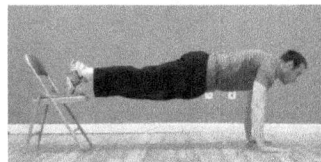 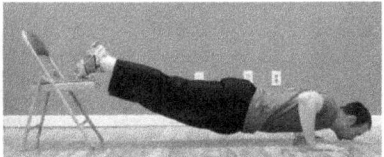

Decline Push Up – Kneel on floor with bench or elevation behind body. Position hands on floor slightly wider than shoulder width. Place feet on bench or elevation. Raise body in plank position with body straight and arms extended. Keeping body straight, lower upper body to floor by bending arms. To allow for full descent, pull head back slightly without arching back. Push body up until arms are extended. Repeat.

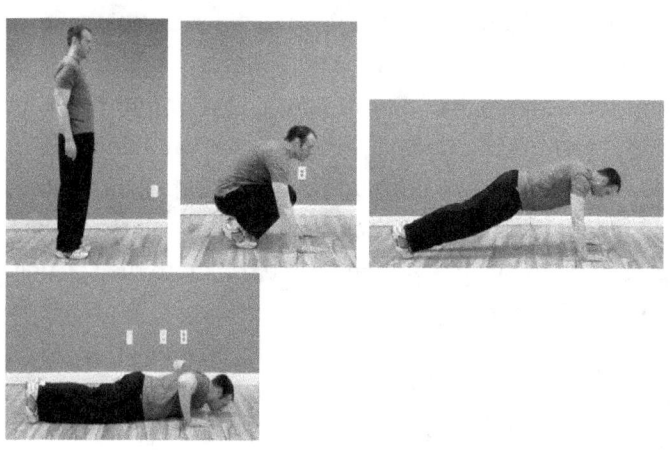

Burpee With Push Up – Start with your feet shoulder width apart. Squat down quickly and place your hands on the floor by your feet kick your legs out until you land in a standard push-up position. Do a normal push-up then jump to your feet and squat backup. This whole exercise is done quickly. Repeat.

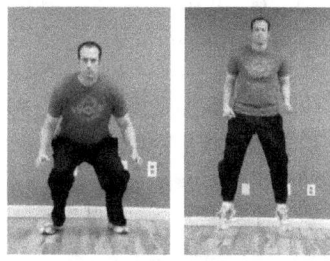

Jump Squats – Begin by standing upright with your feet shoulder-width apart. Keeping your torso erect, slowly bend your legs and allow your body to sink down to a "seated"

position. When your thighs are parallel with the ground, reverse direction and propel yourself into the air as high as possible. Land in an upright position, bending your knees slightly to absorb the shock to your lower body.

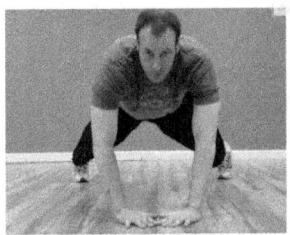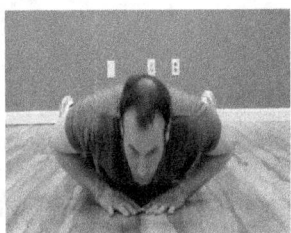

Diamond Push Up – Start in plank position with your hands under your shoulders, and your body in one straight line. Separate your feet so they're about shoulder width apart to help you stay balanced throughout the exercise. Place your hands together, directly under your sternum, with the tips of your index fingers and thumbs touching. Your fingers and thumbs should form a diamond or triangle shape. Bend your elbows out to the sides, and lower your chest toward the floor. Exhale and push back up into starting position.

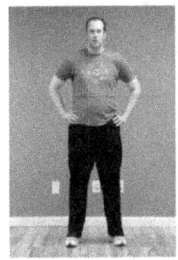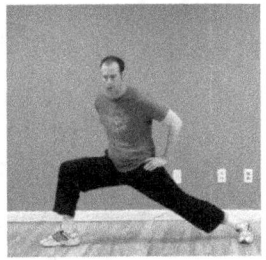

Side To Side Lunge – Lunge to one side with first leg. Land on heel then forefoot. Lower body by flexing knee and hip of lead leg, keeping knee pointed same direction of foot. Return to original standing position by forcibly extending hip and knee of lead leg. Repeat by alternating lunge with opposite leg.

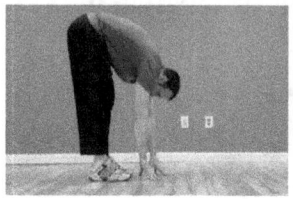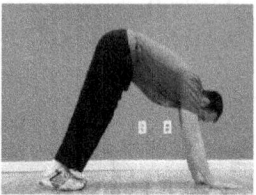

Inchworm – Stand with your feet shoulder width apart and place your hands on the ground in front of your toes. Your knees can be bent slightly the main point is not to get a stretch your hamstrings but to build strength in your upper body. Slowly walk your hands out away from your body shifting your weight onto them. When you get about 2-4 feet or so in front of you slowly walk your hands back toward your feet. Repeat.

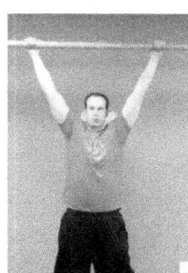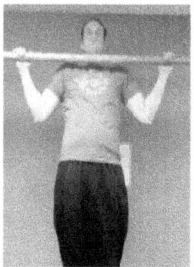

Wide Grip Pull Up – Begin by taking a wider than shoulder-width, overhand grip on a chinning bar. Allow your arms to fully straighten so that you feel a complete stretch in your lats. Bend your knees and cross your ankles over one another. Keeping your back arched, slowly pull yourself upward until your chin rises above the level of the bar. Contract your lats and then slowly lower your body back to the start position.

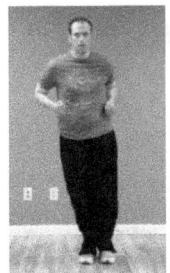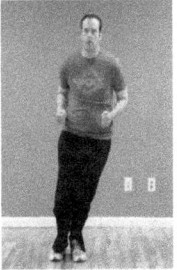

Ski Hops – Jump a short distance from side to side, landing on both feet. Perform exercise at a continuous fast pace.

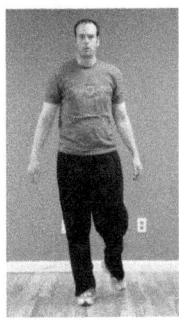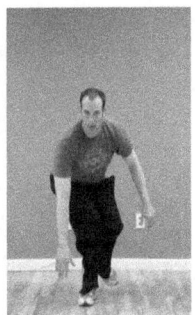

Deadlift Squat – In the start position, lift your right foot off the floor and hold your arms out in front of you. Lower your torso towards the ground while extending your right leg behind you and leaning forwards reaching for the floor. Return to the start position. Switch legs after 8 reps.

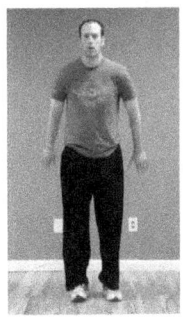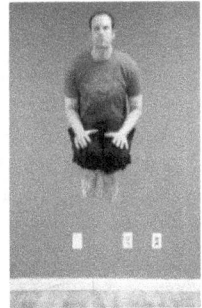

Jump Knee Tuck – Stand with your feet about hip width apart. Begin exercise by getting down into a half squat position and exploding off the ground while bringing your knees as close to your chest as possible. Swing arms upward as you explode off the ground. Try to land softly on the balls of your feet with a bend in your knees and then immediately explode back up. Repeat.

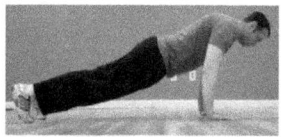 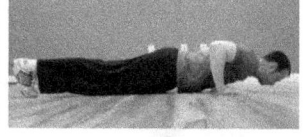

Military Push Up – Place hands directly beneath your shoulders while keeping your arms and elbows tight against your sides. Perform with same movement as Standard Push Up.

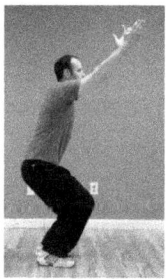

Chair Pose – Stand and raise your arms in front to shoulder height. Contract your arm muscles. Exhale as you bend your knees (no more than 90 degrees) and keep them over your toes.

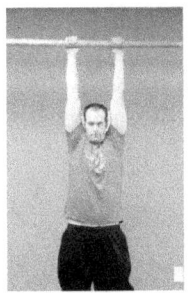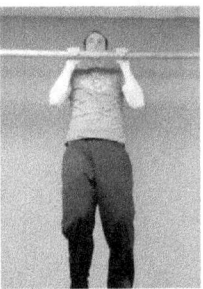

Close Grip Pull Up – Begin by taking an overhand grip on a chinning bar with hands approximately 12 inches apart. Allow your arms to fully straighten so that you feel a complete stretch in your lats. Bend your knees and cross your ankles over one another. Keeping your back arched, slowly pull yourself upward until your chin rises above the level of the bar. Contract your lats and then slowly lower your body back to the start position.

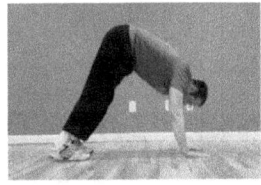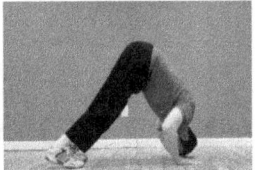

Pike Press – Position your feet wider than shoulder-width apart, and then lean forwards so that you rest your upper body on your outstretched hands. Slowly lower your head towards the ground between your hands while keeping your back and legs straight. Once it's almost touching, push back to the start position.

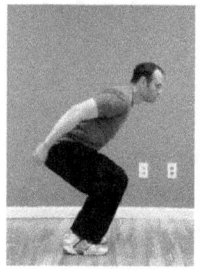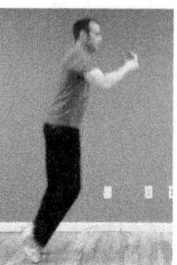

Broad Jump – Place your feet shoulder width apart with your toes lined up. Swing your arms a bit and get your body ready for takeoff. Lean forward slightly, and bend your knees to a bit above parallel. Explode up and out with your legs and swing your arms forward.

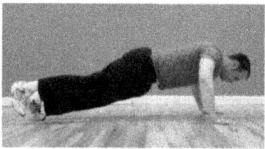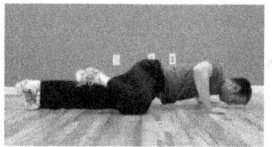

Spiderman Push Up – Get in a normal pushup position. As you lower your body down to the ground lift one knee up and touch the knee to your same side elbow. As you push back up, you bring the leg back to starting position. Repeat on the other side.

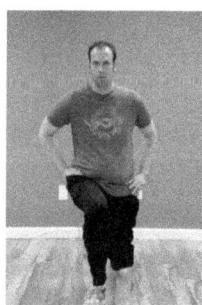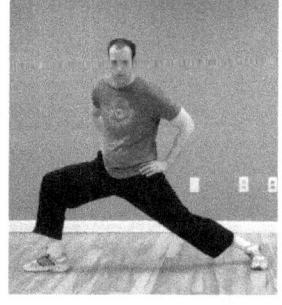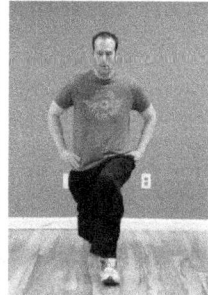

3 Position Lunge – Step forward with right leg. Land on heel then forefoot. Lower body by flexing knee and hip of front leg until knee of rear leg is almost in contact with floor. Stand on forward leg with assistance of rear leg. Lunge forward with opposite leg. Return to standing position and lunge to the right, return to standing position and then lunge to rear. Return to standing position and lunge with left leg forward, to the left, and to the rear. Repeat sequence alternating legs.

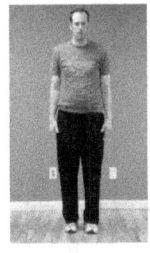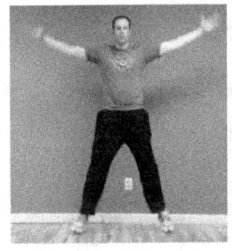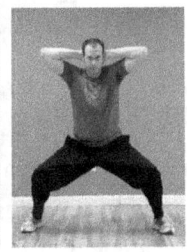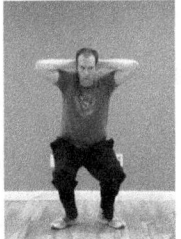

Squat Jack – Start standing with your hands at your side. Begin a regular jumping jack, extending your legs out to the side and arms over your head. After 2 regular jumping jacks place your hands lightly behind your head (as you would in a crunch), but continue moving your legs. Lower your upper body so that you are in a semi-squat position. Continue moving your legs in and out, but just in a constant lowered state.

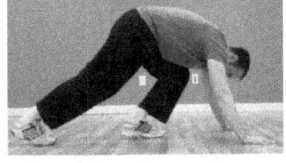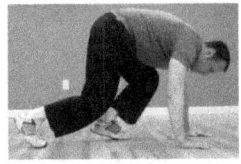

Bear Crawl – In order to properly perform a Bear Crawl, place your hands on the ground about 3 feet in front of you. Keep your buttocks high in the air. Step forward with one of your hands. Then step forward with the opposite foot. Step forward with the other arm and then the other foot. Continue forward in the manner. When you get to the end of the room you can either go backward or turn around and go the other direction.

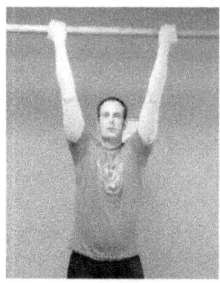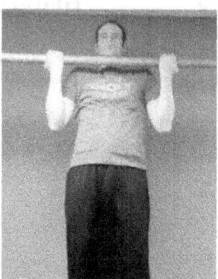

Reverse Grip Pull Up – Begin by taking a shoulder-width, underhand grip on a chinning bar. Allow your arms to fully straighten so that you feel a complete stretch in your lats. Bend your knees and cross your ankles over one another. Keeping your back arched, slowly pull yourself upward until your chin rises above the level of the bar. Contract your lats and then slowly lower your body back to the start position.

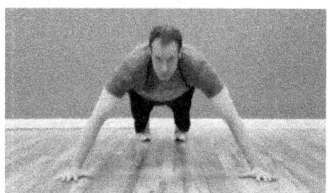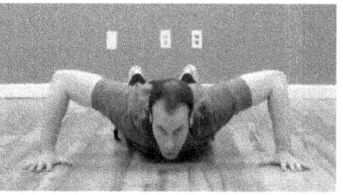

Wide Push Up – Begin with your hands and toes on the floor with your hands placed wider apart than standard push up placement. Your torso and legs should remain rigid, keeping your back perfectly straight throughout the move. Bend your arms and slowly lower your body downward, stopping just before your upper chest touches the ground. Feel a stretch in your chest muscles and then reverse direction, pushing your body up along the same path back to the start position.

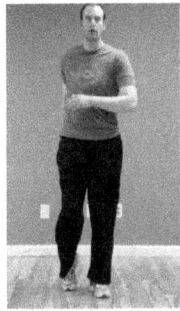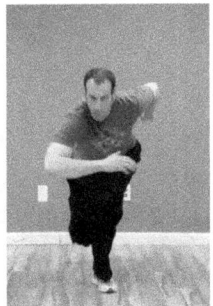

Super Skater – Place all weight on one leg while sliding your other leg behind you with a skating motion. Return back to starting position and repeat for 8 reps and then switch legs.

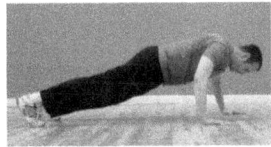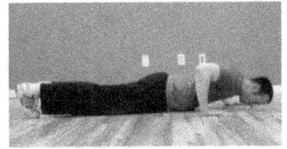

Staggered Hand Push Up – Place one hand in standard pushup position and your other hand a few inches farther forward. Bend your arms and slowly lower your body downward, stopping just before your upper chest touches the ground. Feel a stretch in your chest muscles and then reverse direction, pushing your body up along the same path back to the start position. Switch hand positions after 8 reps.

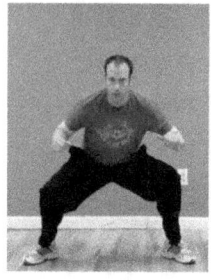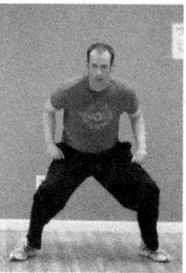

Lateral Leap Frog Squat – Get in a squat position with your legs in a wide stance and your toes pointed outward. Keep your arms forward for stability. Side step to the right by bringing your left leg in first, then your right leg out. Sidestep back to center by bringing your right leg in first, then putting your left leg out.

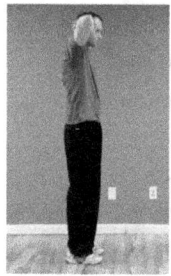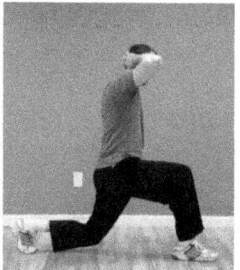

Prisoner Lunges – Stand with your feet shoulder-width apart and clasp your hands behind your head. Keep your elbows pulled back and your shoulder blades should be pulled together to work the upper back. Step forward with your left leg, taking a slightly larger than normal step. Be sure to keep your right toe on the ground and use it to help keep your balance, and also bend your right knee. Continue to lower your body until your front thigh is parallel to the ground. Keep your upper body upright throughout the entire movement. Push with your front (left) leg to return to the starting position and swap legs.

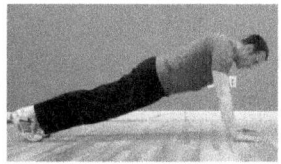 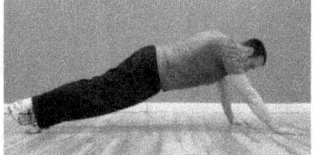

Walking Push Up – Assume a standard push-up position. Hands should be placed on the ground directly under your shoulders. Legs stretched out straight behind you with toes on the ground. This is the starting position. Begin exercise by bringing your right hand and right foot forward about 6 inches and then drop down into a push-up until your chest is just off the ground. Explode back up and then bring your left hand and left foot forward all in one motion and drop back down into a push-up and repeat.

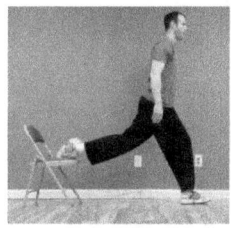 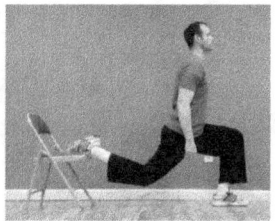

Single Leg Chair Lunge – Extend leg back and place top of foot on bench. Squat down by flexing knee and hip of front leg until knee of rear leg is almost in contact with floor. Return to original standing position by extending hip and knee of forward leg. Repeat for 8 reps. Continue with opposite leg.

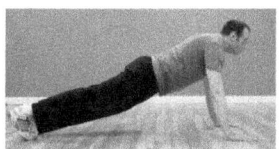 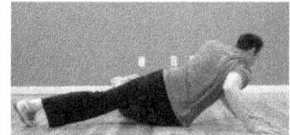

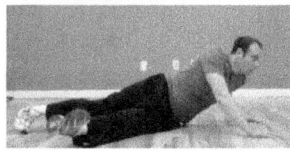

Grasshoppers – Get in a standard push-up position swing your right leg up in underneath you kicking your foot out. Then swing it back and bring it to the starting position. Then repeat on the opposite side.

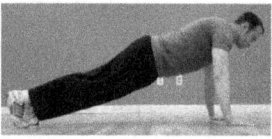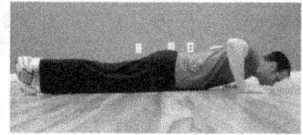

Slow Push Up – Perform standard push up in a slow controlled manner. Take 5 seconds to go down to floor and 5 seconds to come back up and repeat.

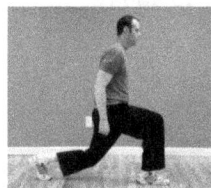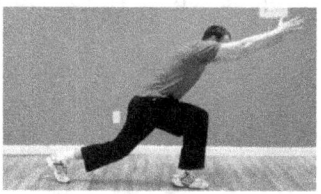

Lunge and Reach – Perform a forward lunge. In the deepest part of the lunge, reach arms anteriorly and parallel (at chest height) as far as you can, maintaining balance. Push back to your starting position and repeat on opposite side.

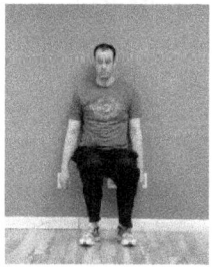

Wall Squat – Stand in front of a wall (about 2 feet in front of it) and lean against it. Slide down until your knees are at about 90-degree angles and hold, keeping the abs contracted, for 20-60

seconds. Come back to start and repeat, holding the squat at different angles to work the lower body in different ways.

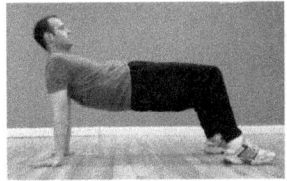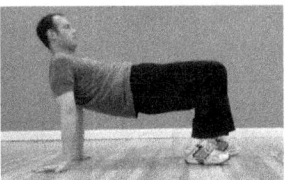

Crab Walk – In order to do a Crab Walk correctly, sit on the ground with your legs extended out in front of you. Place your hands by your side with your fingers pointed toward your feet. Lift your body up into the air. Arch your back up as far as you can making sure your glutes are tight. Now in this position, begin to step forward one hand after the other. As you walk don't let sure butt slump down. When you get to the end of the room turn around and go the other direction.

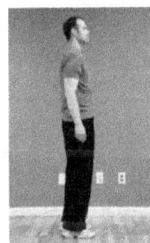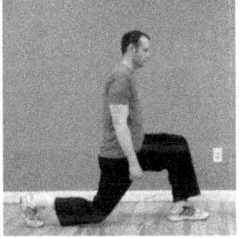

Step Back Lunges – Stand with your feet together. With one foot, take a large stride back and bend both knees to 90 degrees. Using both legs equally, return to the standing position. From there you can alternate and step back using the other leg, or you can perform all the reps on one side and then switch.

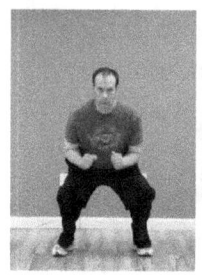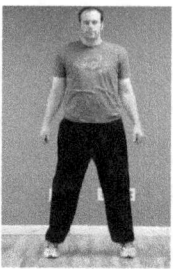

Calf Raise Squats – Stand with your feet shoulder width apart. Move your body into a squatting position while keeping your back as straight as possible. Continue squatting as low as you can until your knees are bent at 90-degrees. Do not go any lower. Stand back up into the starting position. Stand on your toes as you move past the starting position and hold for one second. Return to the starting position.

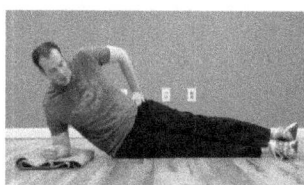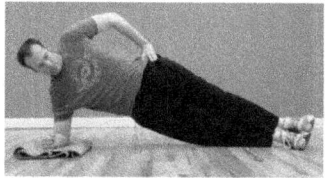

Side Plank – Place your right elbow on the ground. Position your upper body so it is straight and perpendicular to the ground. Place your other hand on your opposite love handle. Hold this position for as long as you can. Repeat on the other side.

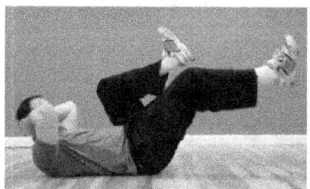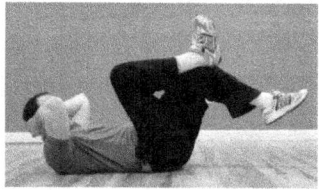

Bicycles – Begin by lying on the floor with your legs bent at a 90-degree angle. Ball your hands into fists and place them at your ears (not behind your head!). Slowly bring your right knee up toward your left elbow and try to touch them to one another. As you return your right leg and left elbow to the start position, bring your left leg toward your right elbow in the same manner. Continue this movement, alternating between right and left sides as if pedaling a bike.

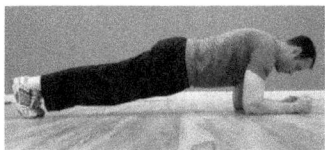

Plank - Lie on your stomach, with your forearms on the floor, your feet together, and your spine in a neutral position. Lift your body up on your palms and toes, keeping your head, torso, and legs in a straight line. Maintain this position for as long as possible. Challenge yourself to maintain the plank position longer each time you perform it. Note: This is a static exercise: no movement should occur once you assume the correct position.

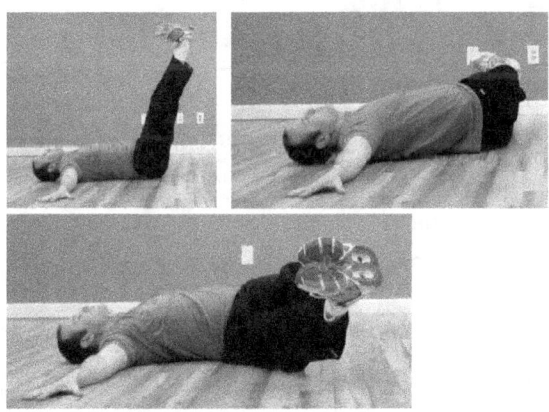

Windshield Wipers – Lay on the ground with your arms out wide. This is to help with balance. Keep your knees straight while lifting them high into the air. Slowly lower your legs to one side until they are close to the ground. Lift them back to starting position and repeat on the other side.

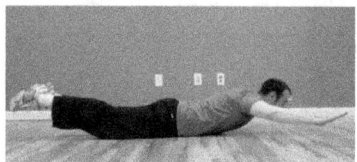

Superman – Lie facedown on the floor, holding your legs together, your arms straight and extended forward, and your head and neck in a neutral position. Keeping your midsection stationary, simultaneously lift your arms and thighs up toward the ceiling to form a soft curve with your body. Contract your glutes, slowly reverse the direction, and return to the starting position.

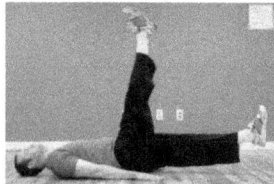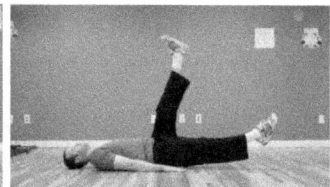

Scissors – Lay on the ground with your hands by your sides. Lift one leg up off the ground while bringing the other leg straight up as if you are forming an L with your legs. Hold for 10 seconds, then bring them together and cross them over each other. Bring them out again and cross them over each other making sure each leg gets a turn being on top.

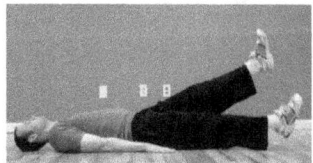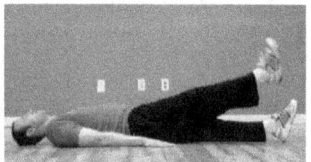

Flutter Kicks – Lay on the ground. Place your hands underneath your buttocks to support your low back. Lift your legs up until your feet are about 3-4 inches off the ground. With your legs straight, begin to alternate lifting one leg higher and then lowering it again.

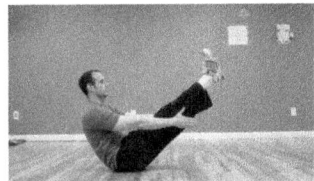

Boat – From a seated position, bring the legs straight up to a 45 degree angle. The torso will naturally fall back, but do not let the spine collapse. Make a "V" shape with the body. Bring the arms out straight in line with the shoulders. Hold position.

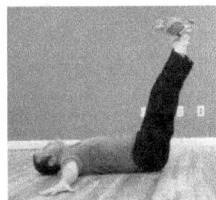 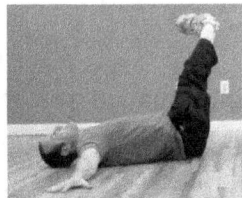 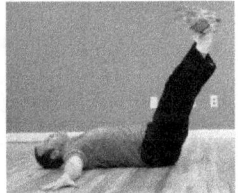

Torso Twist Hold – Lay on the ground with your arms out to the sides, Lift your legs and tilt them side to side at a 45 degree angle. Hold for 30 seconds switch, repeat.

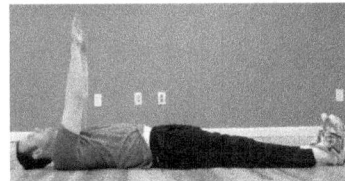 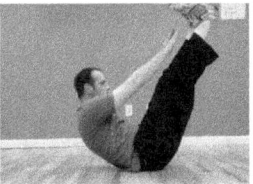

V-Up – Lay face up on the ground with your legs extended and arms above your head. Simultaneously lift your arms and upper body along with your lower legs (knees straight) up until they meet above you. Lower your body and legs back to starting position. Repeat.

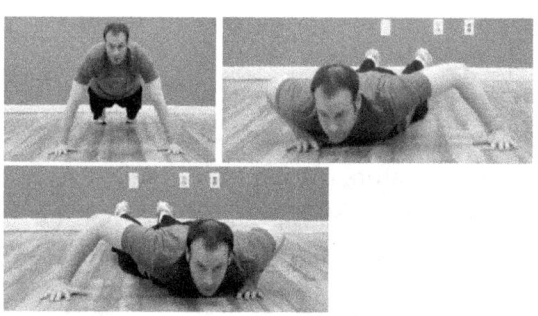

Side to Side Push Up - To perform a side to side pushup what you must do is on the way down for a pushup instead of going straight down the center you should go down towards your right hand. Then when you are at the bottom of the pushup you will be looking directly at your right hand. Now you will move your head and upper body over to the left so you are looking at your left hand and push yourself up. For the second rep you will go down towards your left hand and then over to the right and up again.

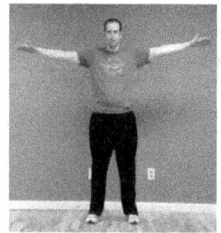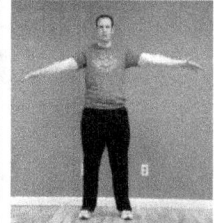

Arm Circles – Stand up and extend your arms straight out by the sides. Slowly start to make circles of about 1 foot in diameter with each outstretched arm. Continue the circular motion of the outstretched arms for about ten seconds. Then reverse the movement, going the opposite direction.

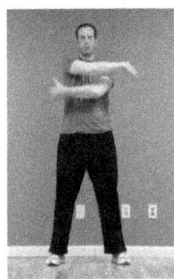 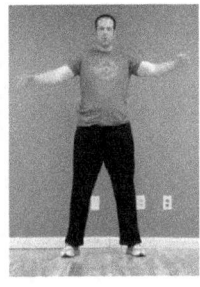 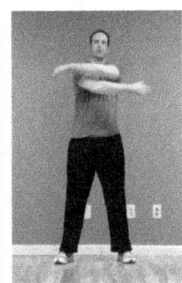

Huggers – Swing your arms like you are giving yourself a hug. Alternate your arm position every 15 seconds.

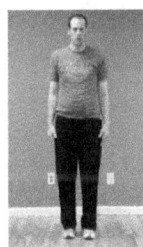 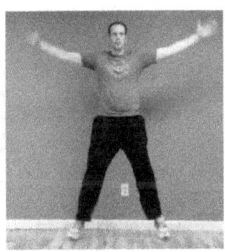

Jumping Jacks - Begin by standing with your feet together and arms at your sides. Bend your knees and jump, moving your feet apart until they are wider than your shoulders. At the same time, raise your arms over your head. Stay on the balls of your feet and be sure to keep your knees bent while you jump again, bringing your feet together and your arms back to your sides. Repeat movement.

www.ingramcontent.com/pod-product-compliance
Lightning Source LLC
Chambersburg PA
CBHW070339290526
45791CB00003B/1396